*Stop the Devil From Laughing When **You** Diet*

You can control your weight
(and other areas of your life) by
mastering the art of resisting
temptation!

Daniel Wychor

Also by Daniel Wychor

Stop the Devil from Laughing When You Diet Journal

"Or didn't you realize that your body is a sacred place, the place of the Holy Spirit? Don't you see that you can't live however you please, squandering what God paid such a high price for? The physical part of you is not some piece of property belonging to the spiritual part of you. God owns the whole works. So let people see God in and through your body."
1 Corinthians 6:19-20 (The Message)

"Education is useless without the Bible. The Bible was America's basic text book in all fields. God's Word, contained in the Bible, has furnished all necessary rules to direct our conduct."
--Noah Webster (1758-1843) -- "The Schoolmaster of the Nation."

Foreword

Years ago a young man sat in his high school class. Boredom set in and he started to doodle. The doodle turned into a picture, why he drew it only God knew.

Some days he drew more than one, sometimes he could go weeks without drawing. He thought they were just to occupy time... but God had a plan.

Four years go by. This young man's father is struggling with overeating. He exercises regularly but keeps gaining weight, and it isn't muscle. He fears that someday his poor eating habits will cause him to have a heart attack while working out. He prays a simple prayer, begging God for help. He thought his prayer was just for him... but God had a plan.

The father is me; the young man my son Alek. What God revealed to me allowed me to break my addiction to binging on junk food and overeating in general. I did not change the foods I eat, with God's help I no longer overeat. I did not give up junk food, with God's help I no longer binge on junk food (yes, it is possible to eat just one). I even exercise less and lost over 20 pounds of fat. My amount of body fat reduced from what doctor's rate as average to ideal.

That however, is not the best part. I have changed from the inside out. The weight cannot return because I am a different person. I now experience the everyday presence of God and temptation does not have the power over me it used to.

I knew as I was undergoing this change that God expected me to use what I learned to help others. What God revealed to me (including using some of Alek's sketches) became this book. This book, along with the program and numerous articles/videos are helping thousands of Christians worldwide resist temptation.
Resisting temptation, that's what this book is about. Whether you just want to stay at your current weight, lose a little or a lot, this book can help you. In just minutes a day you can begin to take back your life. There is an added benefit. While this book deals with weight loss, what you learn can be used to resist temptation in other areas of your life as well.

I was inspired to write what I call an action guide. (I can't stand lengthy books where when I'm finished reading I feel overwhelmed and don't know where to start). While you can finish this book in one sitting, you don't have to read the whole book to get started. You'll find nuggets within chapters that can help you right away. Hopefully you'll be like readers of the original digital version that found the book not only inspired them, but became a resource they could return to at any time.

Use what you learn to develop an awareness of the everyday presence of God. It will amaze you how much more enjoyable your life can become. Along with becoming better at resisting temptation, your life can change in ways that are indescribable.

God bless.

Dan

Table of Contents

Introduction

You cannot win if you don't know you're playing.

The devil is constantly tempting us. He knows our weaknesses and how to exploit them. He knows how to get into our thoughts.

He watches as we have a little success in losing weight. He bides his time knowing if we have some success, and then fail, we'll be more upset than if we had not lost any weight at all. He is waiting for just the right time to tempt us. He already knows what temptations will work; he's used them before with great success. **He just waits and laughs**.

How many times have you dieted and failed? How many times has he laughed at you?

This action guide can show you how to stop him.

Weight loss is a game. On one team are your sinful nature and the devil, which influences you. On the other team is your spiritual nature. Your team is short a player, it's two vs. one, and you wonder why you keep losing.

There is a superstar player watching the game. He would love to play on your team; all you have to do is ask

9

him. If you let him play, and use the abilities he has given you, you win, if you don't, you lose.

"Lean on, trust in, and be confident in the Lord with all your heart and mind and do not rely on your own insight and understanding."
Proverbs 3:5 (Amplified Bible)

As a child I was taught to love Jesus with all my heart. I, like most Christians, however, was not taught how to love him with all my mind. **The battle with the devil is in our minds, not our stomachs**. We allow the devil to influence how we eat without even realizing it. Once we win the battle in our minds, weight loss is a foregone conclusion.

We have been told to focus on God, but not taught how. If we had, there wouldn't be so many overweight Christians.

If you don't learn how to love God with your mind your thoughts become the devil's playground. You cannot give your heart to God and your mind to the devil and expect to be successful.

Imagine being able to control how much you eat and when. Imagine being able to resist the temptation to overeat or eat junk food.

This is not a diet book, it doesn't tell you what to eat and when. It focuses on the ingredient missing in most diets and shows you how to "add" this ingredient. What is this missing ingredient? **God.**

Wonder why you have trouble with your weight? Wonder why you can lose some weight but can't keep it off? You have been fighting supernatural forces, (the devil), on your own and look where it has gotten you. The devil is an expert at temptation. Our trying to fight him alone is like a toddler who just learned how to walk, running in the Olympics. It makes no sense. We need to fight supernatural forces (devil) with supernatural forces (God).

"We use powerful God-tools for smashing warped philosophies, tearing down barriers erected against the truth of God, fitting every loose thought and emotion and impulse into the structure of life shaped by Christ."
2 Corinthians 10:5-6 (The Message)

This is an action guide the devil really hates. It makes you aware of what the devil is doing to your life and gives you moment by moment strategies to thwart the devil at every turn. Once you learn how to use these strategies, you will actually have fun in this game as you realize the devil's temptations don't affect you like they used to. Your thoughts will no longer be the devil's playground.

In the game of weight loss the devil is always playing. You can't expect to win if your best player (God) only plays on Sundays.

Think about that. A lot of people only let God play on Sundays. Many of them let him play only for an hour on Sunday. In fact, many are so preoccupied with other thoughts that they don't even let God play while they're in church!

This action guide will teach you a whole new way to think before, while, and after you eat that can help you lose weight, keep it off and get closer to God all at the same time. Boy, won't that really upset the devil.

After reading this, your perspective on weight loss will change. As you use what you learn, you'll realize that winning the game of weight loss is an opportunity given by God to grow and mature in your faith.

Anyone who struggles with weight can benefit. It also is ideal for families with children. I believe the growing problem of childhood obesity can be stopped by teaching our children some of the strategies outlined in this action guide.

While our focus here is weight loss, there is a wonderful side benefit. Our lives are not just about eating. The devil tries to disrupt other areas of our lives as well. Once you are aware of how he operates, and begin to take action against him, his influence over you will decrease dramatically.

"I say then: Walk in the Spirit, and you shall not fulfill the lust of the flesh."
Galatians 5:16 (NKJV)

1

The Game of Weight Loss

Go team go!

Weight loss is a game. It is a game most people do not win because they do not have a game plan; they have no idea how to play the game to win.

Your enjoyment of playing a game increases when you become good at it. You become good at it by developing certain skills critical to that game, and practicing those skills.

This action guide will teach you skills critical to the weight loss game. As you practice them, they'll become a part of your daily life. When they are part of your daily life, you'll have mastered the game of weight loss, and it will become fun!

How can losing weight be fun? When the devil's temptations don't have the affect on you they used to. **The devil is constantly tempting you. He is not real creative, however.** He keeps using the same moves over and over. Once you know how to counter those moves and keep in game shape (practice) he can't win. You will even find it humorous when he pulls the same old moves over and over again.

In any game, if your goal is to win, you must have a game plan. If you watch any sporting event you'll hear talk of a game plan on each side. If you don't have a game plan, why should you be surprised when you lose?

A game plan is clearly spelled out in the Bible. God has given us a game plan and offered his super natural help. If you play by his rules and let him help, you will surely win.

Just as in any game, there are small battles that must be fought throughout the game. We win some and we lose some. We know the goal is to win the game. We also know that the only way we will win is to stay focused on each battle as it presents itself. As we win battles we get closer to our goal. **One battle is not the entire game.** If we lose a battle the game is not over, we need to put it behind us, learn from it and refocus, ready for the next battle. It is critical that we keep this fact in mind. **We must not throw away today.** If you binge at a meal or snack don't fall into the trap of thinking you can blow the rest of the day and start over tomorrow.

"The reason why many fail in battle is because they wait until the hour of battle. The reason why others succeed is because they have gained their victory on their knees long before the battle came...Anticipate your battles; fight them on your knees before temptation comes, and you will always have victory."
Reuben Torrey Archer

The opponent is the devil. He has a game plan that he has perfected over thousands of years. He doesn't care if you lose some weight, he just doesn't want you to win the game and reach your goal. He knows most people will win some of the battles but lose the game. He'll be happy because they'll be more depressed than when they started. He's real happy with people who just give up after playing the game several times and losing some battles. "The devil made me do it" is truer than you think. Each battle in the game of weight loss is a battle with the devil. Those of us who struggle with our eating habits are in a battle with the devil every time we eat.

It is important as we play this game that we see ourselves not through our eyes but through God's eyes. God loves us for who we are and knows what we can become.

God knows the unique gifts he has given each one of us and what we can do. He is just waiting to see if we will ask for his help and do it. We only know ourselves for who we are. We focus on our limitations, God focuses on our possibilities. In looking through God's eyes, we will focus on what we can become.

God plays many roles in this game. He is the owner watching the game from the owner's box. He provides us with all that we need to play the game. He is the coach giving us words of wisdom and motivating us. He is the star player we can call on to help us win the game. God (the owner) has given us a valuable piece of equipment that we must use properly to win the game. That equipment is your ability to imagine. We must train our imagination to focus on God and what is good, not what is bad.

The devil knows he cannot win if you train your imagination to focus on God and what is good.

The devil is very skilled at planting bad seeds in our minds. If you find yourself in a continual rut you can't seem to get out of there is a simple reason. You are allowing those bad seeds to grow into negative thoughts. You are continually imagining negative things, things not working in your favor. **There is no way to get out of that rut until you learn how to get rid of those bad seeds before they can grow.** *You need to learn how to use your imagination to focus on God and what is good.*

"Don't judge each day by the harvest you reap ... but by the seeds you plant!"
Robert Louis Stevenson

God says if you pray and believe something will happen before it does, you will receive it. We do this by praying, believing and then imagining (or visualizing) winning battles before the actual battles take place.

You visualize many times during the day without realizing it. **A visualization can last for minutes or a microsecond.** When you day dream you are visualizing. When you have a negative thought, you are visualizing. Anytime you are afraid to do something, or don't believe you can, it is because you are visualizing (or picturing in your mind) ahead of time that you will fail. If you are not afraid to do something it is because you are visualizing you will be successful. Often this is because you've already been successful at it before.

An example of visualizing is planning a vacation. You gather literature, make travel plans, and get time off work. You haven't gone on the vacation yet, but you believe you will be. You even visualize the fun you will have and you haven't even left yet! Visualizing has been proven in numerous studies to increase success, whether it is in athletics, business, school or everyday life.

Another example is a study done years ago at the University of Chicago. The study was done to determine if visualizing could affect the free throw performance of basketball players.

First, the athletes were tested to find out how well they currently shot free throws. They were then placed at random in one of three groups.

The first group went to the gym everyday and shot free throws for one hour.

The second group also went to the gym but did not shoot free throws. Instead, they lay down and visualized themselves shooting free throws, with every shot they visualized going in the basket.

The third group did nothing. They were told to not even think about basketball.

After 30 days, the three groups were once again tested to find out how well they shot free throws. The results were amazing! The players in the group who did nothing showed no improvement, in fact many did worse.

The players in the group that practiced one hour each day showed an improvement of 24 percent.

Now here's the amazing part, the group that just visualized, did nothing but imagine shooting free throws, improved 23 percent! That's right, **the group that did nothing but imagine shooting free throws did almost as well as those that practiced!**

If you keep failing, part of the reason is you continually visualize failing without even knowing it!

I enjoy reading articles about successful people and what it is they do that makes them successful. A common thread among many who excel is:

1) They are consistent in how they approach a challenge, (they approach the challenge the same way each time).

2) It starts in the mind – what they think about and visualize before their big event is critical to their success.

3) They are able to stay calm and focused throughout the challenge.

Let's do a little experiment. I will give you some words and you see what comes to mind. The words are black and white cow.

What came to mind? For most people a picture of a black and white cow came to mind. The reason for this is we think in terms of pictures, not words. When we think of someone or something, a picture flashes in our mind. It may happen where we are consciously aware of it or it may happen in a microsecond.

What does this mean? Whether you are aware of it or not, **every time you have a positive or negative thought, you picture that positive or negative thought.** Just like the basketball study, if you are constantly having positive thoughts, you are picturing yourself being successful, and your success rate will improve.

On the other hand, if you're constantly having negative thoughts you are picturing yourself failing and you will fail more often. This is the scenario the devil loves, he knows he has you and is slowly devouring you.

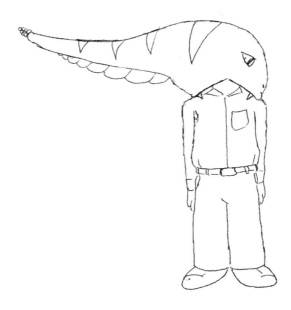

Throughout this book you will be given various visualization exercises that if you start to use on a regular basis, will totally transform your thoughts. You will learn to focus on God and stay focused, so as battles come up, you are ready. **As you do the visualizations it is important to imagine them from the perspective of the**

first person. You are in it, not watching it happen like a movie.

Do not do them while operating any equipment or driving. It is ideal if you can do them in a quiet setting where you can relax and not be disturbed.

This book is being interrupted for a brief message.

Studies show many people do not read beyond the first chapter when they buy a book. If you are thinking of stopping at this point, (guess who put the thought in your head to quit), **THE DEVIL WILL KEEP LAUGHING!** *He does not want you to continue, he knows if you continue and use what you learn, his influence over you will decrease dramatically!* ***It's Your Choice.***

Now, back to the book.

"All Satan's Apples Have Worms. I do not deny that the Devil has some pretty apples; I just say that all of them are fakes and that after you bite into them, you will find they have worms. All Satan's apples have worms."
John R. Rice

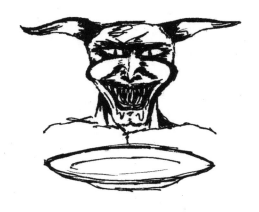

2

The Opponent

The Tempter himself.

I remember hearing of a study done a few years ago that asked people a simple question, "Do you believe the devil exists?" The results were very interesting. More than 2/3 of those surveyed, whether religious or not said they believed the devil existed. Of those who considered themselves very religious, more than 80 % said they believed the devil existed.

So most people believe the devil exists, but few think about the effect he could be having on their struggles with weight. Why is that so? Is it because they can't see him?

What would happen if we looked at other things we cannot see the same way?

We can't see the wind. If we didn't account for the effect it has on us what would happen? Boats would struggle getting to their destinations because of the wind effects on currents and sails. Airplanes would struggle with not only getting to their destinations but on take offs and landings.

We can't see gravity. What would happen if you ignored the effect gravity has on you? Do you think you might struggle in your daily life? After a few broken dishes or broken bones I'd say you'd start taking it into account.

If you believe the devil exists, wouldn't common sense tell you that you should start considering the effect he could be having on your weight loss struggles?

Let's take a closer look at our opponent.

As I stated before, **the devil is an expert in temptation.** One of the names used for him in the Bible is "The Tempter." He has been tempting man since Adam and Eve set foot on earth. How can we even think that we have a chance of resisting his temptations on a regular basis without help from God?

I've heard some people say that they didn't believe the devil has anything to do with people struggling with weight. Their argument is that there are a lot of people who do not struggle with weight or are able to lose weight and keep it off on their own.

My simple comeback is he doesn't use food exclusively as the only temptation. I know of many people who have never really struggled with their weight. When you take a close look at their lives you'll find he tempts them in other ways. Some are heavy smokers, some have a drinking problem. Others have had drug issues and the list goes on and on. The point is he tempts us all, just not all in the same way. In fact, we all have more than one area of our lives where we struggle with temptation.

Now back to those who struggle with weight…

What did the devil use in his first temptation of man? Food. He knows eating is pleasurable. I believe the devil gets a lot of enjoyment out of toying with us when God is not in the picture. Have you ever been depressed and tempted? Have you ever been extremely hungry and tempted? Have you ever been distracted by other things and tempted? The devil knows that without God, our weak sinful nature will give in, and the devil loves every minute of it.

"Don't assume that you know it all. Run to God! Run from evil! Your body will glow with health, your very bones will vibrate with life!"
Proverbs 3:7-8 (The Message)

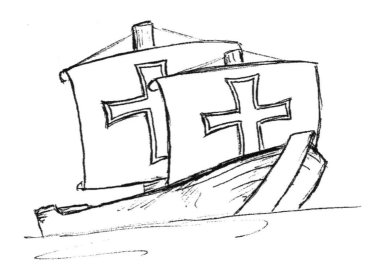

3

Where Did God Go?

He was here a minute ago.

You sit down to eat this delicious meal; the aromas are making you hungrier by the second. All you can think about is how good this food is going to taste. But first you must say grace. As you say "amen" and pick up that fork any thoughts of God are gone. All you can think about is FOOD---NOW! Where did God go?

You are having donuts after church in the fellowship hall. You bite into that donut in God's house, are you thinking of him? You are shopping for groceries with temptation all around you, are you thinking about God?

You are standing with the fridge or pantry open staring into it, trying to decide what you want to eat, whether you're hungry or not. Are you thinking about God?

You are out to dinner staring at the menu trying to decide what to order. Are you thinking about God?

What if you turned eating into a spiritual experience? What if you kept God front and center in your mind before you decide what to eat and while you were eating.

Would that change how you look at food? Would that change what you ate on a regular basis? Could you lose weight and keep it off?

Along with whatever diet or eating plan you are on, what if you allowed God to be your personal weight loss counselor and used the Bible to be your weight loss guide?

Many preachers say man works in the natural whereas God works in the supernatural. Do you think if you allowed God to use his supernatural powers to assist you in losing weight you'd be more successful than you have been on your own? Do you think it's at least worth a try?

Think about God OFTEN.

"Is prayer your steering wheel or your spare tire?"
Corrie Ten Boom

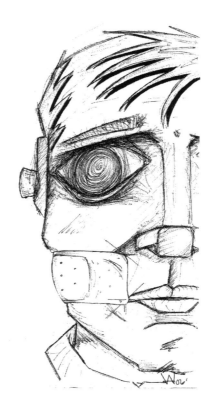

4

Food Zombies

How did that food jump in my mouth?

Most people who have weight problems are what I call food zombies. If you ever saw any of the old horror movies, you'd see these bodies staggering around and it appeared nobody was home upstairs. The brain was not functioning.

I used to be a food zombie. I'd walk in the kitchen and the common sense part of my brain would shut down. I'd think about what I wanted to eat or just grab something when tempted. I'd then continue eating until I ran out of what I was eating or became so stuffed I couldn't eat another bite. I'd walk out of the kitchen and voila! My brain turned back on. The first thought was, why did I do that? I felt lousy physically, and mentally started beating myself up. Then I'd swear I was not going to continue to eat like this anymore.

This continued day after day, week after week, month after month, year after year.

Do you remember the story of the Israelites leaving Egypt and wandering in the wilderness for 40 years? They were afraid to enter the land God had promised, they feared it was inhabited by giants. I was watching Joyce Meyer on her TV show Enjoying Everyday Life®. She said they spent forty years wandering for what should have been an eleven day journey. She said that only two of the approximately two million who started the journey went into the Promised Land, the rest were descendants. The two who God allowed to enter thought differently than the rest, they did not see giants but a land flowing with milk and honey.

Most people spend their entire lives as food zombies walking in what I call the "weight loss wilderness". They end up seeing weight loss as a giant they fear they cannot conquer. Those who believe and trust God and allow him to help can get out of this wilderness. They will enter the Promised Land where their temple is fit and trim as God designed it. The length of the journey will differ for each person, depending on how much weight they need to lose. Whether its weeks or months, the Promised Land will be reached by most within one year. And then they will be home, NO MORE WANDERING!

It's important to note at this time that we operate on God's schedule, not our own. Some people lose weight faster than others. Don't get hung up on how fast you lose the weight. Focus on the process and you will reach your goal in the time God wanted you to.

"Dear friend, guard Clear Thinking and Common Sense with your life; don't for a minute lose sight of them. They'll keep your soul alive and well, they'll keep you fit and attractive."
Proverbs 3:21-22 (The Message)

5

God's Temple

"Or didn't you realize that your body is a sacred place, the place of the Holy Spirit? Don't you see that you can't live however you please, squandering what God paid such a high price for? The physical part of you is not some piece of property belonging to the spiritual part of you. God owns the whole works. So let people see God in and through your body."
1 Corinthians 6:19-20 (The Message)

Would you store cases of dynamite in the church sanctuary? How about tons of toxic garbage? Would you take a bag of garbage with you to church on Sunday and dump it on the altar? What a horrible thought, no way!

Your body is God's temple. By gorging on food day after day without thought, that is exactly what you are doing. You are creating an explosive, toxic situation in your own body, God's temple.

Think about this for a moment. The Holy Spirit is in you. Your body is a temple.

I was watching Dr. Frederick K.C. Price (Ever Increasing Faith Ministries®) one Sunday and he put it another way. He talked about how people will abuse their bodies (smoke, do drugs, overeat etc.) outside of church, but wouldn't consider do those things in the church. He used as an example people who smoke on the way to church and put out the cigarette before entering the church. Why? Because they respect it as a house of God. They believe it is a holy place.

I have a news flash for you…God says your body is a temple, this means your body is a holy place! **YOUR BODY IS A HOUSE OF GOD, THE BIBLE SAYS SO**. Why then, do we treat our bodies differently than the physical church we attend? I believe it comes down to awareness. If we are always aware of the Lord's presence, we won't abuse our temple as we may have in the past.

Imagine walking into the fellowship hall after church to enjoy some refreshments and conversation. You walk up to the table and gaze at the variety of choices available to you. Donuts, rolls, coffee cake, coffee, juice, heroine, cocaine, whiskey, vodka. What!

The donuts, rolls and coffee cake are just as deadly to an overweight person as the drugs are to an addict and alcohol to an alcoholic.

If you are overweight and enjoy the after church fellowship, have someone get your juice or coffee for you and stay as far away from the table as possible. If you must eat, bring something nutritious with you. If you can't leave the sweets alone don't go. Some will say they so enjoy the fellowship and I understand. However, if we are to bring pleasure to God in all we do we need to find ways for fellowship without destroying his temple. **Do**

you think God would be pleased if we had a fellowship meeting in the church and dumped bags of garbage in the church while we met?

Are you addicted to certain foods? Are there foods that if it is available to be eaten you have to eat it? I have always had this problem with sweets. If I see it I will eat it and usually not stop until I've gorged on it. I set up a rule in my house that if sweets came in the house I did not want to see them, they were to be hidden. This worked great until I started to crave sweets and went looking for "hidden treasure". I'd find the hidden goodies and binge. I did not think it was right to deny other family members who did not have a weight problem and could eat sweets in moderation so I came up with a solution. I bought a lock box that required a key to open it. I don't have a key so I can't get at the sweets.

If you live alone there is no reason for foods you are addicted to being in the house. I believe God will help in any area of our lives but he expects us to do our part and take the first step.

When it comes down to it, we were created by God, we did not create ourselves. **Our bodies are on loan from God**. He has made us caretakers of our bodies. The American Heritage Dictionary defines caretaker as "a person employed to look after or take charge of goods, property, or a person." In other words God has given each of us a body (temple) to look after. If a friend asked you to look after her house while she was on vacation, what would you do? Would you throw wild parties and trash the place or watch over it with care. You have a choice and I'm willing to bet 99% of you would watch over it with care.

God has given each of us a temple to look after. We do have a choice as to how we care for it. 99% of us are willing to look after a friend's house with care, yet most of us are not willing to show that same care toward God's temple.

Your Body IS God's Temple - Take Care of It!

"If you have no joy, there's a leak in your Christianity somewhere."
Billy Sunday

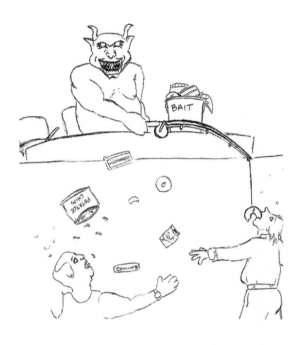

6

Success

Are you really good at overeating?

You are already successful when it comes to weight. Say what? You have become very successful at gaining weight. You had to consistently overeat day after day for a long period of time to get where you are. You have actually trained yourself to overeat and/or eat junk food. **You actually visualize doing it, without even knowing it.** But you have not done this alone. The devil tempts us constantly and instead of being aware of what he is doing we think we are just weak and have no control. If we do try to resist the temptation we go it alone.

Here is a simple question, who is more powerful, the devil or God? If we ask for God's help and also do our part, do you think God will respond? With God's help can you defeat the devil?

Imagine how you'll feel knowing God is helping you when tempted. Imagine him helping you to consistently eat healthy day after day for a long period of time?

Imagine what that will do for you not only physically but mentally.

You are soon going to learn some very easy ways to do this and become very successful at losing weight and more importantly, keeping it off.

"A person without self-control is like a house with its doors and windows knocked out."
Proverbs 25:28 (The Message)

"There are good days and there are bad days, and this is one of them."
Lawrence Welk

"The vigor of our spiritual life will be in exact proportion to the place held by the bible in our life and thoughts."
George Mueller

7

Here's Jesus!

Think about Jesus while you eat.

In chapter one I asked you, "where did God go?"
Hebrews 3:1 says "Fix your thoughts on Jesus. 2
Timothy 2:8 says "Always think about Jesus
Christ." It doesn't say only when we pray, only in
church or Bible study, it says ALWAYS. Most people
aren't thinking about Jesus when they think about food
and start eating. They say a prayer just before eating and
as they reach for the fork all thoughts of Jesus are gone.
Most people rarely think of Jesus when they reach for a
snack. The more we focus on Jesus, the easier it is to win
the game of weight loss.

We are told over and over again to put God first in our
lives but we weren't told how to do it when we eat. Is it
any surprise so many are overweight?

Focus your thoughts on the presence of God.

"God can do anything, you know – far more than you could ever imagine or guess or request in your wildest dreams! He does it not by pushing us around but by working within us, his Spirit deeply and gently within us."
Ephesians 3:20 (The Message)

8

What God Revealed to Me

It's all about the nourishment.

I am one of those people who actually enjoys working out (it's lucky I enjoy it, I had a serious back injury years ago that forces me to stay in shape. If I don't work out for a few days I begin to experience complications from the injury). I work out at least 4 days a week, around 1 hour per workout.

A typical day of eating for me would go like this. I would win the battle at breakfast and usually at lunch. I would lose the snack battle before dinner, lose the dinner battle and lose the snack before bedtime battle. Depending on the day the score was either Devil 4, me 1 or Devil 3, me 2. I was worried if I kept on this path that some day I'd be one of the guys that died young of a heart attack during their intense workout. I would try to eat right but my gorging habits would take over consistently night after night. I tried everything under the sun and did great for a short while and then would fall back into my old habits. I finally reached my wits end and prayed to God to please help me.

"Let go and let God." That's the thought that came into my head and then he gave me the following revelation. I was to take the emotional intensity I experience when I eat the host at communion and apply it to every bite I eat. When I am given the bread, the body of Christ at communion, I look at it closely, noticing its texture and then put it into my mouth. I savor this precious food, feeling its texture in my mouth and its flavor. Knowing what has been given to me makes this a very intense experience.

The next time I sat down to eat I picked up a fork full of food and studied it. Something miraculous then happened that made it more intense. The words, "Thank you Lord, for this nourishment" came out of my mouth. I had not planned on saying anything, it just came out. I ate the food with the same intensity of communion and it was amazing. The food tasted better and I savored it much more than I usually do. I was no longer eating on auto pilot. I continued to do this with each bite, studying the food, thanking the Lord and savoring it. It was the most intense meal I had ever experienced. I also was eating slower, feeling much more satisfied and surprise, ate less!

I wondered why he put the word nourishment in my little prayer instead of food. I don't use the word nourishment in my everyday vocabulary. Then it hit me, the word food applies to anything edible whereas nourishment applies only to foods that are good for you. I began to find myself avoiding junk food because I couldn't pray that prayer before eating it. Awesome!

Use the word nourishment in place of the word food when you eat healthy.

"Trust in the Lord with all your heart and lean not on your own understanding; in all your ways acknowledge Him, and He shall direct your paths."
Proverbs 3:5-6 (NKJV)

"The scriptures are given not to increase our knowledge, but to change our lives."
Dwight L. Moody

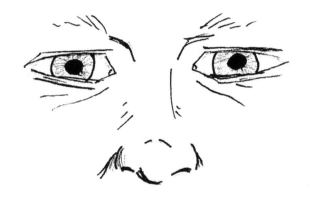

9

Learning to Focus on Jesus

Feed your mind and the body will follow.

W e get caught up in the little things in life and worrying about what others think about us yet we rarely think about he who controls the whole universe! He wants to help us but he won't force himself on us. He'll tug at our heart strings to suggest how to get on track but we often ignore his advice, and we wonder why we have problems! How can we develop a constant focus so he is in the forefront when we make even the most mundane decisions?

How did you get good at the things you like to do? To be a good athlete in any sport you have to practice. To be a good singer, dancer, painter etc. you have to practice. To focus on Jesus at all times you have to practice. But how do I do that?

"Start with God – the first step in learning is bowing down to God; only fools thumb their noses at such wisdom and learning."
Proverbs 1:7 (The Message)

Start by reading the Bible. I find I get much more out of each reading if I approach it with a hunger, an eagerness of what God will reveal to me next. I say a small pray before I start that God will reveal something special to me in this reading. If you approach it like you do when you read a book you can't put down, you'll get a lot more out of it. Set aside time each day, preferable the same time, so it becomes a habit. I like to read a chapter in the morning and one in the evening just before I go to bed. Make sure as you are reading that you are not distracted by other thoughts (again, the devil at work). Stay focused on what you are reading. If you can afford more than one Bible, own a variety of translations. The way a certain verse is translated in one may make more sense to you than another.

Read books by religious people. Let them act as mentors in helping you deepen your faith. There are many out there who have devoted their lives to studying God's word and can provide valuable insights.

Listen to Christian radio. The uplifting talk and music will help you stay focused on Jesus. Just focusing on the lyrics to the songs can provide you with new insights.

Listen to tapes/CD's from various ministries. There is a lot of good material on a variety of topics.

Watch Christian TV. Unless you're watching a must see show you'll benefit more from hearing and seeing God's word.

I cannot overemphasize how important it is for you to guard carefully what you allow into your mind.

Your subconscious will absorb like a sponge anything you focus on. If you listen to or watch anything negative on a regular basis it will affect you and keep you from your best.

Most everyone who was raised in a Christian church has a certain way they are used to hearing the word of God delivered to them. I was raised in a conservative church where other than singing the hymns or reciting prayers we sat quietly and listened. I was very uncomfortable with churches where people had more of what I call a whole body experience during their worship, praising God during the message, dancing and swaying during hymns, etc. I believed that everybody had a way they were comfortable in worshipping and I was content to stick with my way. Then one day I turned on Christian TV to see what was on. It was a service where the preacher was hollering, the people were shouting and my mind was screaming, "turn the channel!" I could not do it. Something inside me said, "**Focus on the message, not the messenger**." It was hard but I did it and my eyes were opened. I began to step out of my comfort zone and watch TV services and preachers I would never have watched before. Each time I did, God planted in the message something important he wanted me to hear. I call these God's gems, his "diamonds in the rough." I now watch with anticipation anytime I turn on Christian TV to see what gems God has in store for me.

Don't be afraid to watch preachers who have speaking styles that don't appeal to you. Focus on the message, not how it is delivered. You never know when God is going to present you with gems of information.

I have heard the Holy Spirit within each person referred to as the seed of God. By reading God's word and hearing about him you are watering and fertilizing that seed. The more time you spend the more the seed begins to grow in you. You begin to notice positive changes in your life and in the way you think. You'll begin to feel a calming presence coming over your life. You'll still have everyday problems to deal with but you won't feel like you're in it alone.

Practice the visualizations in this action guide on a regular basis. How would you feel about the start to your day if right when you wake up you imagine Jesus standing at the foot of your bed smiling at you saying, "Wake up, I made today, let's be happy and enjoy this day!"

Does change happen overnight? For some it does, but for most it's a gradual process. You must have the mind set of a farmer, who plants seeds and patiently cares for them. He knows that even though he sees nothing now, eventually he'll have a bountiful harvest. He has complete trust in the process and you must too.

You might be thinking, "When am I going to find time to do this?" If you're channel surfing you've got time to watch Christian TV. If you're reading the news in the newspaper or on the internet you've got time to read God's word. Besides, it's healthier for you to read the positive message of God than the negative message of the media.

**"Test all things: hold fast what is good.
Abstain from every form of evil."**
1 Thessalonians 5:21-22 (NKJV)

**"Therefore submit to God. Resist the devil and
he will flee from you."**
James 4:7 (NKJV)

10

Resistance

Do this, not that.

I believe the devil is very good at getting us to resist doing what is right. Obviously he is going to work overtime planting bad thought seeds in our minds when something we do will get us closer to God.

Think back to the last chapter. Do you resist reading the Bible daily? Do you resist watching Christian television? Do you resist listening to Christian music? Do you resist reading books by Christian authors?

Think about what you do read on a regular basis. Think about what you watch on a regular basis. Think about what you listen to on a regular basis. Does what you read/watch focus on positive or negative ideas? Are they bringing you closer to God or further away? If your answer is further away, it should come as no surprise you don't feel in control of your life.

"And all things, whatsoever ye shall ask in prayer, believing, ye shall receive."
Matthew 21:22 (KJV)

"And whatever you ask for in prayer, having faith and [really] believing, you will receive."
Matthew 21:22 (Amplified Bible)

11

Visualization

What you see is what you get.

Your brain can't tell the difference between what is real and what is imagined. Everyone has fears that are only imagined, but to them are real. As discussed earlier, if we visualize certain things that will help us in our weight loss; our brain will perceive them as real.

I had one Christian try to claim that visualization was not biblical. In John 4:35 (King James Version) Jesus said to his disciples, "Say not ye, there are yet four months, and then cometh harvest? Behold, I say unto you, lift up your eyes, and look on the fields; for they are white already to harvest."

The fields were not ripe; they were four months away from being ready. The only way they could "see" what Jesus saw was to visualize.

God has given us a wonderful gift in our body and our mind. Think back to Chapter One when I showed you through the black and white cow exercise how your mind thinks in pictures, not words. It is important to remember that every time you have a thought, whether it is good or bad, you are visualizing.

Please read again the verses just before this chapter. They are the same verse, just different translations. What they are saying is to receive what you pray for, you must believe it's a done deal; you must act as if you have already received what you have prayed for.

This is a hard concept for a lot of people. How do you believe to the point where you act as if you already have received? I believe this is why God gave us the ability to visualize. Think back to the basketball study. Those that just imagined shooting free throws did almost as well as those that actually practiced. There mind perceived the visualizing as real. When tested a second time their body reacted as if they had actually been practicing.

We are going to start getting into various visualization exercises. Before we start I want to make an important point. The more detail you add to each visualization, the more real it will appear in your mind and the more effective it will be in helping you.

Let's use the basketball study again as an example. The players visualizing went into amazing detail. They imagined walking up to the free throw line. In their minds they could see and feel the basketball in their hands (they may have even noticed the smell of a leather basketball). Some imagined bouncing the ball and hearing it hit the floor before they shot. They looked at the basketball hoop, noticed the color of the metal, texture of the net. When they shot the ball they imagined it flying towards the hoop and going into the net.

When you do the visualizations, add as much detail as you can.

Let's do a quick exercise. I want you to think of a loved one, it can be a person or a pet. As you visualize this person or pet add as much detail as you can. What does their hair or fur look like? Is it combed or messy? What color is it? Look at their eyes. What color are they? Look at their teeth. Are they straight or crooked, white or discolored? What smell if any do you associate with this loved one? If a person, what are they wearing? Notice the color and texture of the fabric. If a person, imagine them saying "I love you" and listen closely to the sound of their voice. If a pet, imagine the sound they make when they are happy to see you. Imagine hugging this loved one. Please do this exercise now.

You'll find the more senses you involve; sight, sound, touch, smell, feel, taste, the more intense the visualization and the more effective it will be.

When we get into later visualizations that involve the devil, add as many negative characteristics to him as you can. Give him bad breath, horrible body odor, scaly skin, whiny voice, the works. If he is offering you food, it doesn't hurt to imagine it is spoiled and has a bug or two crawling on it.

When you visualize Jesus, see him in all his splendor. You want to have the feelings for him in your visualizations that you did for the loved one we visualized earlier.

The more contrast you make between Jesus and the devil the more effective the visualization.

Are you ready? Let's get started.

Try this visualization.

Go into your kitchen and find something healthy to eat, like a piece of fruit. Set it on the counter in front of you.

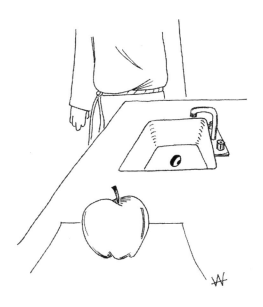

Imagine Jesus is standing in front of you. He is smiling at you like a parent smiles at his/her child. Look into his eyes and see all the love he has for you. Notice everything you can about him. The lines in his face, his hair, his clothing etc. Pick up the fruit. Look at it closely, noticing its texture. Smell the fruit and enjoy its fragrant aroma.

Look into his eyes and say as if this was the only food you would eat today "Thank you Lord, for this nourishment."

Turn away and set the fruit down. Pick up the fruit again and do it again. Repeat this 10 times.

After you have done this, go over to your cupboard and pick out some junk food. Set it on the same spot on the counter that you had the fruit.

Imagine Jesus standing in front of you just as before. Pick up the junk food. Look at it closely, notice its texture and smell it. Think about what this junk food will do to your body once you have eaten it.

Look into his eyes and say, "Thank you for this nourishment." Were you able to do this? As I started to reach in the cupboard for junk food my hand recoiled, I couldn't touch it, let alone pick it up. The more intense your visualization of Jesus the more likely you are not to want to touch the junk food.

Why is that? I believe it comes from our wanting to please God, to care for his temple. We know instinctively that putting junk food into our body does not bring him pleasure. We as Christians are taught from a young age that God wants us to be good.

Try this visualization next time you eat a meal.
Imagine you are with Jesus and the 5000 when he fed them the fish and bread.

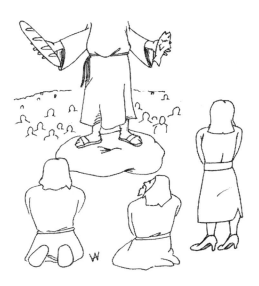

Feel the warmth of the sun on your skin, notice the smell of the water nearby. Feel the refreshing breeze in your hair.

Imagine the food you are eating was miraculously prepared by Jesus.

Look around you and notice other people in the crowd. As you eat each bite, look at Jesus and thank him for the nourishment.

Did you get into the visualization? If you did, wasn't it amazing? If you didn't, remember, someone is trying to distract you from getting closer to God. Give it another try.

Visualization – Jesus at Your Table

Imagine Jesus sitting across from you, watching as you eat. Look at him closely, the loving look in his eyes, his beautiful smile etc.

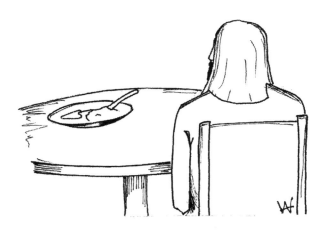

After each bite, look at him and say, "thank you Lord, for this nourishment."

If I am at home, I'll say it out loud, if I am eating out, I'll say it softly to myself or in my head.

I found it helpful when I first started doing this visualization to pull a chair away from the table as I would for someone else. If you do this before you eat it will remind you of what you are to do. To add more detail, visualize Jesus walking over, sitting down and thanking you for moving the chair for him.

"The shortest distance between a problem and a solution is the distance between your knees and the floor."
Charles Stanley

Visualization- At the Lord's Feet

The following visualization is really powerful, it can be extremely intense (It is hard for me not to cry every time I do it, but I love this visualization). You may want to do this in private. It alone can create an intense desire to want to care for your body. If you are able to, do this visualization kneeling.

Imagine you are kneeling at the foot of a cross.

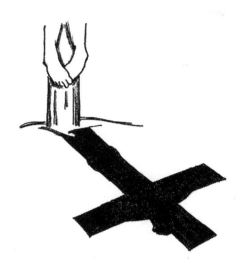

You are so close to the cross you can touch it. You notice the grain in the wood and how rough the cutting is. You reach out and touch a sliver of wood that is sticking out from the cross with your finger. It is so sharp it pricks your finger.

Your gaze now shifts up the length of the cross. Looking down at you is Jesus, dying on the cross. You can see everything, the spikes in his feet and hands, the crown of thorns. You hear his labored breathing, and see the blood coming from his wounds. You look at his face and see sweat on his chin. Your gaze moves up his face and you see where the thorns are piercing the skin on his forehead. You can see droplets of blood forming on the thorns that pierce his skin.

You drop your head and gaze at the ground. A droplet of sweat from his chin lands on the back of your neck.

You look up again and Jesus is staring at you with his piercing eyes, they seem to look right through you. The look on his face is a combination of pain and love… for you. He says, "I am doing this, for you, take care of my Father's temple named (your name) for me."

You respond, "I will take care of this temple, my Lord and Savior, Jesus Christ."

Visualization – Waking Up

This is a great visualization to do each morning as soon as you wake up, while you are still in bed.

Imagine you just woke up from a good nights sleep. You look at the foot of your bed. Standing there is Jesus.

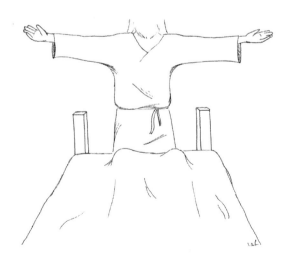

His clothing is radiant; it's as if the sun is shining behind him. He is looking at you with a beautiful loving smile. His eyes sparkle. He stretches his arms out to you and says, "I have made this day, let's be happy and enjoy it!"

"For by your words you will be justified, and
by your words, you will be condemned."
Matthew 12:37 (NKJV)

"Words are powerful; take them seriously.
Words can be your salvation. Words can also
be your damnation."
Matthew 12:37 (The Message)

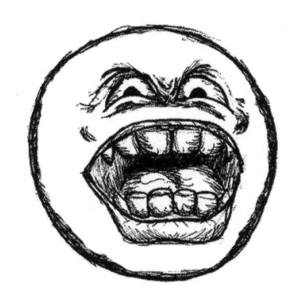

12

The Power of Your Words

Out of the mouth of babes, and adults too.

Y ou are well aware of how your words can affect other people in a positive or negative way. Let's take a closer look at how they affect you.

We discussed earlier how when you have a thought your mind sees a picture, positive or negative. What you say has the same affect on you. If you are saying negative things, your mind follows with a negative picture. If you say positive things, your mind follows with a positive picture. That's why it is so critical to be careful what you say.

As you can see by the verse above, the Bible is very clear on the importance of words and how they affect you.

Words are clearly important in winning the weight loss game. That is why it is important that you include affirmations as part of your daily routine. Affirmations are positive statements we believe to be true. An example is, "When tempted I will follow Jesus." Bible verses make great affirmations. I recommend memorizing Bible verses and using them along with other positive statements. I have included some at the back of this action guide.

Some people say affirmations don't work. In some cases they are correct. How could that be? If someone is in a negative state and does not believe the affirmation they are saying, what affect will it have? Most likely it will have no effect; they might as well be speaking gibberish. **It is critical that the affirmations you use are ones you believe to be true.**

"Keep my message in plain view at all times, Concentrate! Learn it by heart! Those who discover these words live, really live; Body and soul, they're bursting with health."
Proverbs 4:21-22 (The Message)

13

The Devil's Virus

Auto update with God daily for protection.

I was working on my computer one day and it turned out to be infected with a virus. I had a virus scanner scanning the files in my computer, searching for the virus. During this time the virus kept trying to trick me in different ways, pretending it actually wanted to get rid of itself. Pop up windows would appear on the screen, telling me to visit a phony web site that was pretending to be a windows security center. At first I was really shook up as this virus tried to lure me to more trouble. Once I was on to all its tricks, I wasn't worried. I knew it was just a matter of time before my anti-virus software found it and finished the virus off.

It was as I was waiting for the virus scanning to finish, that God revealed something to me. All of the negative thoughts and temptations I experience are no different than the virus in my computer. They disrupt the efficient operation of my life, causing me to waste time and energy. The devil is behind these negative thoughts and temptations. I realized that if I treat each as a devil's virus

I will bring it to the forefront of my thoughts. By immediately switching my focus to Jesus (by visualizing his presence and saying affirmations), I was able to "remove" that negative thought or temptation and get back on track.

It is the little daily thoughts that shape your life. It is critical that when negative thoughts or temptations pop up, you immediately change your focus to Jesus.

We spend money on keeping our computers safe with anti-virus software yet we don't protect our own minds from the devil's "viruses."

We protect the family computer, but we don't protect our minds or our children's minds.

The anti-devil software is God's word. By loading it into your brain and updating it daily you can keep yourself protected. Reading the Bible, watching Christian TV, listening to Christian radio, reading books by Christian authors, bible studies etc. are all anti-devil virus software. Just thinking about God in moments of temptation can be enough to delete the devil's virus.

The more you focus on God the stronger your faith will grow. The stronger your faith becomes, the more God will use his supernatural powers in your life.

I like how Charles Stanley (In Touch Ministries®) phrased the degrees of faith. A person with a weak faith believes "God can." A person with a great faith believes "God will." A person with a perfect faith, a Godly faith believes "It's done."

People with a perfect faith have no doubt. They believe that what they are asking God to do will absolutely happen. I believe these are people who have had miraculous cures or succeeded against seemingly insurmountable odds.

You are no different than them. Continually grow in your faith and allow God to work miracles for you.

"Life becomes harder for us when we live for others, but it also becomes richer and happier."
Albert Schweitzer

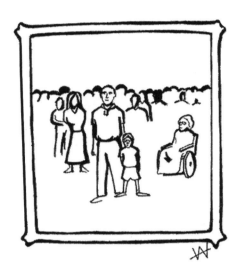

14

It's not just About You

You're always eating for more than just one.

Childhood obesity is on the rise. It's all over the news. Many children are following the examples of their parents and becoming food zombies. If we don't get a handle on it, there will be more young people suffering from health problems caused by obesity than ever in our history.

Children don't do as you say, they do as you do. Look at how you have been letting the devil have his way with you. Look at the example you are setting for your children, **remember they do as you do.**

Imagine your child decades from now experiencing the same problems you are going through. Is that what you want for your kids?

You have a choice. You can make the decision to use what you have learned in this book to let God change the path you are on. You can set the example for your children. Decide today that you will no longer abuse the temple God has given you and teach them to stop abusing theirs. As your children see the tremendous change in you it will begin to have an effect on them.

Imagine the new you your children see, the one focused on Jesus.

What a great legacy to leave your children, showing them how allowing God into every area of your life can set you free.

I would think any parent would give their life to save the life of their own child. When danger is staring us in the face we will do anything to protect our children. Yet, when it comes to their future health we are blind. **If you were told that your child will live one more day if you don't eat a cookie today, would you eat the cookie?** I don't think so.

What would happen if every time you wanted to overeat, you realized that you could be shortening the life of your children?

Would you say to yourself, "they'll live long enough, who cares if they live an extra year or two," or would you say "my children are more important to me than stuffing myself." Could this thought process help you to stop your cycle of overeating? **"It's not just about me."** That statement really helped me begin winning more food battles. I began to repeat it to myself whenever I thought of eating and it kept me in control. Studies have shown we experience more joy when we help others than when we help ourselves. By shifting our focus from ourselves to how others will benefit, or be harmed by how we eat, changes everything.

We get so caught up in ourselves we really don't think much about how our behavior affects others. Do you realize that how you take care of the temple God has given you, can affect not only your children but also your grandchildren and generations to come? We just don't realize how the choices we make in our lives can set the standard for future generations.

I recall hearing of a study that followed the descendants of two different people, one an upstanding citizen, the other a criminal. It was amazing to see over the generations how many of the upstanding citizens' descendants became successful, well adjusted people, whereas the criminal's descendants followed in his footsteps and remained the dregs of society.

How many people do you know who said when they were young, "I'm never going to be like my parents!" Were you one of them? How many of these same people as they got older turned out just like their parents? How often have you heard people say, "I can't help it, my parents were the same way."

Studies have shown that children of overweight parents have a greater chance of being overweight than of being normal weight.

You have an opportunity to not only help yourself and your children but also set the bar for future generations.

Generations from now your descendants may be pointing at you, saying for good or bad they are the way they are because of the example you set.

If that's not enough incentive for you to lose weight the results of a recent study may convince you. A startling new study funded by the National Institute on Aging and published in the New England Journal of Medicine® found that if you get fat, chances are your family and friends will too. The study found the following:

If you become obese, your friends' chances of becoming obese go up 57 percent, your siblings chances go up 40 percent and your spouses chances go up 37 percent. In the case of your closest friends, if you become obese their chances of becoming obese almost triple! The study also found where you live doesn't matter. The chances are the same whether you live next door or hundreds of miles away. Based on the findings, the researchers suggest that obesity is "socially contagious" and can spread easily from person to person. By this point it should be pretty obvious that it's not just about you.

Focus on Jesus and be a shining light for all your friends, relatives and all that follow you.

Visualization – The Mirror (As You Are Now)

Take a good look at yourself in the mirror. Notice in detail the excess weight on your body.

Imagine behind you is your child (ren) as adults, in the same physical shape. Imagine behind your children a line of thousands of people, people as far as your eyes can see, all in the same physical shape as you are.

These are your descendants for generations to come. Statistics say if you do nothing about your temple this is the legacy you will leave. Do you like what you see?

Visualization - The Mirror (Your Temple As God Intended)

Look at yourself in the mirror, not as you are but with the slim fit temple God intended you to have. Notice in detail how beautiful your temple is.

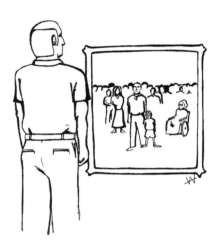

Imagine behind you are your child (ren) as adults slim and fit. Behind them are thousands of descendants all looking slim and fit. They are all smiling at you, thanking you for the example you set for them. You can hear them saying "Thank you (your name)." If you allow God to help you become slim and fit, this is the likely legacy you will leave.

Remember, there are other people that your weight can affect. Friends, other relatives, neighbor kids, co-workers etc. Often we are not even aware of how much influence we have on them. If you want, (or if you don't have children), imagine some of these people in the mirror visualizations, with their descendants standing behind them. It may make the visualizations even more powerful.

"And behold, I am with you and will keep (watch over you with care, take notice of) you wherever you may go..." And He said, "My Presence will go with you, and I will give you rest."
Exodus 33:14 (NKJV)

"Blessed be the Lord, Who bears our burdens and carries us day by day..."
Psalm 68:19 (Amplified Bible)

"Fear not, for I am with you..."
Isaiah 43:5 (NKJV)

"For I am with you to save you and deliver you," says the Lord.
Jeremiah 15:20 (NKJV)

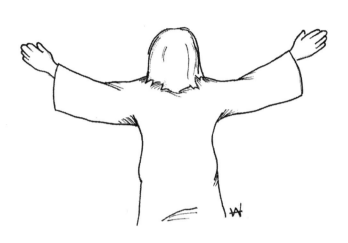

15

Following Jesus

Bring Jesus with you wherever you go.

I have mentioned throughout this book the importance of focusing on Jesus. The bible tells us that God is with us **ALWAYS**. We are told we are to follow Jesus, to be followers of Jesus. You know he is with you right now, this very minute, so how can you keep him in the forefront of your thoughts? First you have to realize that God has given you a choice and most of us keep making the wrong choice. **God is with us always but he will not force himself on us and into the weight loss game.** We must allow him into our lives and when we do we are changed forever.

To maintain focus on Jesus and allow him into your life moment by moment, follow Jesus, **I mean literally follow Jesus!** Remember when I discussed imagining Jesus standing by you or sitting by you while eating? **When I say literally follow Jesus, I mean imagine walking along side him or following him wherever you go.** If Jesus is walking with you wherever you go, do you think you might start making better choices in all areas of your life?

As I was grocery shopping one day I was thinking about how I could keep my mind focused on Jesus. The thought came into my head, "let me push the cart." If anyone was looking at me they must have wondered what happened, I must have had a shocked look on my face. I thought no, I can't visualize Jesus pushing my shopping cart, that's just not right. **The next thought was, "hey, I've washed feet, now let me push your cart!"** I couldn't argue with that. I imagined Jesus pushing my cart as I went through the grocery store (I walked in front of the cart and pulled to give him a hand.) That was the most interesting grocery shopping trip I have ever had.

Visualization – Grocery Store

Imagine you have just entered your favorite grocery store. Guess who will be pushing your shopping cart? **Jesus**.

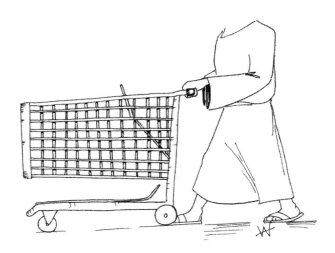

Imagine Jesus telling you how much he loves you and how proud he is of how you are cleaning up your temple.

Imagine walking each aisle of the store and putting the groceries in the cart. As you walk down the aisle that contains your greatest junk food temptations how do you feel? Can you put any junk food in the cart when Jesus is with you? **Do you think the devil is getting a little upset now that you have a new shopping buddy?**

How did you feel on your little shopping trip? Did you find yourself wanting to please Jesus? When I went shopping, Jesus said I could get whatever I wanted; I had the power of choice. I found myself thinking when I looked at a food, "will Jesus be pleased with me if I put this in the cart?"

Try this visualization the next time you actually go grocery shopping. Instead of pushing your cart either walk along side or in front and pull your cart and let Jesus do the pushing. **Training your mind to follow Jesus can change your life.** Allow him to be with you whether you're watching TV, gardening, working around the house, going to a ball game etc. **He wants us to enjoy life and wants to be a part of our lives.** By following him everywhere you'll begin to enjoy life like you never imagined.

"Isn't it obvious that all angels are sent to help out with those lined up to receive salvation?"
Hebrews 1:14 (The Message)

Want to add a little muscle to your visualizing? When I am feeling especially weak I imagine Jesus showing up with the troops. If you are a Christian, you know that God has sent angels to help watch over us and protect us. Why not imagine that a couple of warrior angels in battle gear, each carrying a spear, are with you to help protect you from the devil.

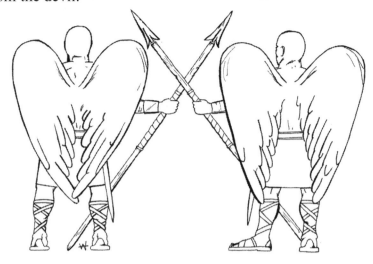

I have used this visualization grocery shopping. One time I was in the cookie aisle staring at some mouth watering chocolate cookies. I imagined the angels stepped in front of me and crossed their spears so I couldn't touch the cookies. It worked; I didn't touch them and went on my merry way.

I am really big on visualizing Jesus because it really helps us to keep him first in our thoughts. You cannot go wrong when you do that. Focusing on Jesus can keep you out of trouble.

Think of Peter when Jesus told him to get out of the boat and come to him. While Peter kept his focus on Jesus he was walking on water. When he looked away at the waves he began to sink.

When you stay focused on Jesus and totally trust in him, he brings his supernatural powers to bat for you. Turn away and you are on your own. Seems like a pretty easy choice to make, yet all too often we forget what he can do for us.

Visualization – Walking On Water to Jesus

Imagine you are standing on the edge of a dock. The surface of the lake is only a few inches from the top of the dock. It's a beautiful sunny day with a few wispy clouds in the sky.

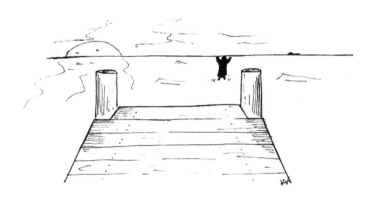

You are looking out across a peaceful serene lake. The water is so still it looks like glass. You can see the reflection of the clouds on the surface of the lake. On the other side of the lake is nothing but woods, it is so beautiful. You can hear the birds singing in the trees behind you.

You look across the lake towards the other shore and see someone standing, yes standing, in the middle of the lake. Standing on the surface of the lake is Jesus. His face is glowing, he has a brilliant smile. His eyes are a clear blue and look as if beams of light are radiating from them. His robe is a brilliant white and his arms are outstretched... towards you. He says, "Gaze into my eyes and come to me."

You focus on his eyes....and step off the dock. You are standing on water! As you start to walk towards him you can feel the surface of the water on the bottom of your feet. You know if you divert your gaze from his eyes you will sink.

This is one of my favorite visualizations. It is fascinating to me the yearning to reach him that comes over me each time I do this visualization. When I first started doing this I would not get very far before I would look at the lake and sink. As I've continued my journey I keep getting closer but have not made it all the way to his outstretched arms.

I was blown away one day while doing this visualization. When I reached a certain point in my walk to him something amazing happened. While gazing into his eyes they began to change! I was mesmerized as I watched them change from the clear blue with beams of light to a deep black with spiraling galaxies in each eye. I have found that each time I have done this visualization since, this change occurs at the same point in my journey to him.

"You've got to be careful if you don't know
where you're going, because you might not get
there."
Yogi Berra

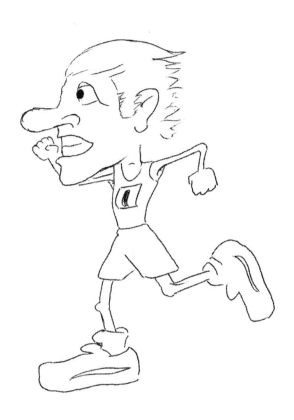

16

Eat Right - Exercise Later

You cannot outrun overeating.

I have always been an advocate of getting regular exercise. It wasn't until recently that I realized I had my priorities wrong. Recent studies have shown that weight loss is approximately 80% eating right and 20% exercise. It is very easy to eat more in calories than your body can burn, no matter how much you work out. I know this to be true from personal experience. I was doing intense workouts at least 4 days a week and gaining in areas that definitely were not muscle.

Gaining weight is not rocket science. If what you eat has more calories than your body burns up, you gain weight. If you exercise and you still eat more calories than you burn up, guess what? You'll gain weight at a slower rate but you will still gain weight. This was me.

I'm sure you are aware of all the information out there on eating the proper foods, not starving yourself. Starving yourself slows your metabolism and that is not smart (although the devil would like you to starve yourself, knowing it leads to failure.) We want to reveal God's temple as he designed it. He didn't design us to be just skin and bones. If you already get regular exercise that's great, I'm not telling you to stop. What I am saying is it's critical that you use what you've learned here to get your eating battles under control. If you don't currently exercise, as you lose weight you'll have more energy and naturally want to become more active. Find physical activities that you enjoy doing, (always check with your doctor first) and have fun. **To win the weight loss game you must think eat right first, exercise second.**

"Dear friend, guard Clear Thinking and Common Sense with your life; don't for a moment lose sight of them, they'll keep you fit and attractive."
Proverbs 3:21-22 (The Message)

17

The Key to Staying Focused

See God all around you.

As God inspired me and I started using what he gave me, I felt like I was on a roller coaster. When I stayed focused I did great, when I lost focus I would binge. As well intentioned as I was, I would find myself slipping back into my old habits. After a day of massive binging, instead of getting depressed I sat down to analyze what I was doing wrong. Following is the list I came up with, see if any of them sound familiar to you.

1- Not listening to spirit suggesting to me what to eat. I often times go into the kitchen to eat a meal and the thought of what I should eat pops into my head. I would reject this thought and start grazing on a variety of foods which usually lead to binging.

2- No plan as to what I wanted to eat. I have found this to be a recipe for disaster for my waist line. More often than not this leads to binging.

3- Thinking about what I want to eat next before I have finished what I am currently eating. Talk about mindless eating, it was obvious to me I was just shoving food into my mouth, not enjoying it or focusing on what I was eating.

4- Experiencing an eating frenzy. I got into a package of cookies for my daughter's lunches. My mind was not on eating a cookie but on eating a whole row of cookies.

5- No focus on what I was doing to my body (God's Temple). I had not given any thought to what I was doing.

6- Not thinking about Jesus. Fact of the matter is I was not thinking about anything. It was as if my body had reverted to act as if famine was right around the corner. It was if I needed to stuff as much food into it as I could to survive.

7- Eating very fast. I was shoving food into my mouth at a frenzied pace. I wasn't taking a bite of the cookie (my rationale was I would get crumbs on myself or the counter), I was stuffing the whole cookie in my mouth and reaching for another before I had swallowed.

8- No self-discipline, completely out of control. Not until I was stuffed and could eat no more did my brain come back on-line and did I think about what I had just done. I remembered my brain trying to interject during the feeding frenzy but I shut out what it was trying to say.

9- Standing while eating. It was real easy to hunt for food while I was still eating the last food. As I read the list I realized this binging was a regular habit in my life. I had to get it under control if I was to succeed at getting God's temple to the size he intended. I realized that I had a habit of becoming a food zombie whenever I am around food.

GOD spoke to Moses: "Speak to the People of Israel. Tell them that from now on they are to make tassels on the corners of their garments and to mark each corner tassel with a blue thread. When you look at these tassels you'll remember and keep all the commandments of GOD, and not get distracted by everything you feel or see that seduces you into infidelities. The tassels will signal remembrance and observance of all my commandments, to live a holy life to GOD."
Numbers 15:37-40 (The Message)

As you can see from the above Bible verse, **God instructed the people of Israel to use awareness cues to remember to keep the commandments of God.** He wanted them to use them to stay focused, so they did not get distracted by their sinful nature and the devil's temptations.

The thought came to me to start using awareness cues to get me back to focusing on Jesus and keep me from becoming a dreaded food zombie. I started putting notes on the fridge, on the pantry that said "focus on Jesus."

While it worked some of the time to snap me out of it, often times I didn't read it (I'd ignore it), so it didn't work. Then a thought came to me.

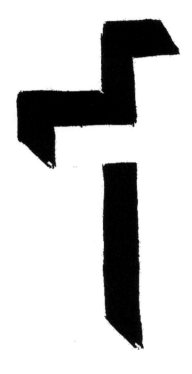

In the movies they often use a cross to ward off evil. I took out a marker and drew a cross on a piece of paper and hung it on the fridge. I did the same on the pantry. Now when I go into the kitchen the first thing I see is a cross and my focus is on Jesus.

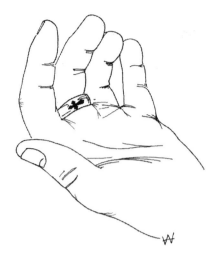

I bought a ring with a cross on it. I wear the cross part of the ring on the inside of my hand. When I look at the palm of my hand, I see the cross on the ring and imagine the wounds in Jesus hands from his crucifixion.

When I pick up something to eat I see the cross on my ring and my focus is on Jesus. In my mind the cross was linked to Jesus and warding off evil. It worked! Hello Jesus, goodbye food zombie!

The more cues you can use to keep you focused the better. I have provided some that work for me. Try coming up with your own cues also and visualize them over and over in your mind. The more you do this, the more ingrained it will become. After a while when tempted in a similar situation, you'll be amazed as it automatically pops up to get you back to focusing on Jesus.

Visualization – Food Choice, Jesus vs. Devil

If you find yourself looking at a choice of junk food and nourishment and you're struggling, try this.

Imagine Jesus and the devil are standing in front of you.

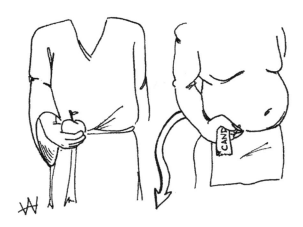

Imagine Jesus is holding the healthy food out to you. He is smiling at you, expecting you to make the right choice.

Imagine the devil is standing next to him holding the junk food out to you. The devil has a sly look and blazing red eyes.

Jesus says to you, "It's your choice."

"Put God in charge of your work, then what you've planned will take place."
Proverbs 16:3 (The Message)

18

Motivation

It's all about the who.

Most people believe that losing weight is a strictly personal experience that only involves their physical body. Their motivation is purely self-centered. If I lose weight I'll look better. It obvious that this belief is not enough motivation for the vast majority of overweight people. If it were, everyone would be in great shape.

"Focusing on the self is the opposite of focusing on God."
Romans 8:7 (The Message)

God did not make us to be self-centered. He wired us to get our greatest enjoyment out of life when we are doing things for others not ourselves. It is when we are thinking and doing things for others, being what I call selfless, that we are at our best. I believe we bring God great pleasure when we are selfless. The most selfless person to ever live was someone named Jesus and we know God was quite pleased with him.

I found one of the keys to winning the game of weight loss is to approach it from a selfless perspective.

As I stated earlier, **it's not all about you; it's about how the change in you will benefit others.** If you give yourself enough reasons why losing weight and keeping it off will please God and help others, it will come off and stay off. Give yourself a big enough WHY outside of you and the weight loss is inevitable.

Instead of thinking ME, ME, ME, begin thinking WHO, WHO, WHO.

Think about many of the things discussed earlier. Think of how setting a great example for your children and how being your best will affect many of your descendants.

Think of how pleased God will be that you are now taking care of his temple like he knew you could. Realize what God is revealing to you is a gift, not only to improve yourself, but to use you as an example for others.

As you play the game of weight loss you will lose some battles. **It is important that you keep in mind at these times not only are you still in the game, but that you are not doing this just for you.** You are doing this for thousands of people here now and yet to come. As you are winning the game you will become closer to God and grow spiritually day after day. We as Christians are told to spread the good news of Jesus Christ. One of the best ways to do this is to be an example to others. As you uncover the beautiful temple God gave you, you'll develop a new way to share the Word.

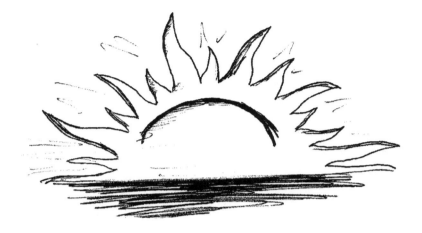

God wants you to shine. He wants you to be a beacon to the world of what it means to be a Christian. As you reveal the temple he gave you, people will notice you have changed inside and out. They will want to know what you know. They will want what you have. **Share**.

**"Temptation usually comes in through a door
that has deliberately been left open."**
Arnold Glasow

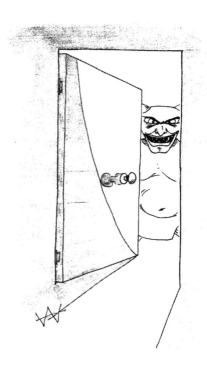

19

No Cracks

Keep that door closed or you'll let in more than a draft!

The devil is not looking for a wide open door to enter. He is looking for a crack. He doesn't give you the thought, "eat half the cake, or eat half the bag of chips. The temptation he gives you is "have a small piece, it won't hurt you, or have just a serving of chips." He knows what your weaknesses are and what foods lead you to binge.

I call these small temptations "cracks." These are the critical thoughts you must guard against, these are the ones that occur over and over and keep you from reaching your goal. You must keep in your mind **NO CRACKS**. You must see them for what they are and not give in. **Knowing that these cracks turn into a wide open door is half the battle.**

"The devil loves 'curing' a small fault by giving you a great one."
C.S. Lewis

Time for an exercise. Get a pencil and paper. Make a list of those foods that you crave and have a habit of binging on. Think back over the past months when you've had these foods in the house. Remember when you ate those foods, what was your first thought when you saw the food? Write down the thought you had just before you ate each food. We are not looking for exact words, just the general idea. Do this now.

Did you think, "I want to really pig out on this food and eat at least 1000 excess calories?" I doubt it. When I did this I found I was thinking the same thoughts over and over. "Just a small piece, only a few, just a small dish, only a spoonful, were common." These were foods I had a history of binging on, foods I was addicted to. I foolishly thought I could control urges without making any changes in my life.

"The definition of insanity is doing the same thing over and over and expecting different results."
Albert Einstein

We are doing the same thing over and over when we allow the devil to get to us through these cracks. It's time we realized this and started doing things differently.

Visualization – Devil Food Fight
Imagine you are standing in front of your pantry. Focus on a package of whatever food you craved most recently.

What was the thought that convinced you to starting to eat that food? Does this same thought come to mind each time you are going to eat something you shouldn't?

Imagine picking up some of this food in your hand.

To your side is a door that is open just a crack, the devil is looking at you through the crack. He is sneering at you and laughing. Imagine throwing the food and as it splatters on the devil's face say out loud with a firm voice, **"NO CRACKS!"**

The more detail you add to the visualization the better it will work. Imagine the food really made a mess of the devil. Imagine it running down his face and as he looks at you with a shocked look, have a good belly laugh.

Repeat this with each food you crave.

"Yet the Lord is faithful, and He will strengthen [you] and set you on a firm foundation and guard you from the evil [one]."
2 Thessalonians 3:3 (Amplified Bible)

"Now that we know what we have – Jesus, this great High priest with ready access to God – let's not let it slip through our fingers. We don't have a priest who is out of touch with our reality. He's been through weakness and testing, experienced it all – all but the sin. So let's walk right up to him and get what he is so ready to give. Take the mercy, accept the help."
Hebrews 4:14-16 (The Message)

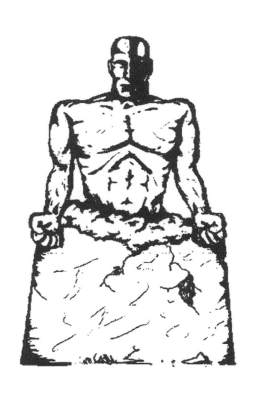

20

When the Temple is Revealed

So this is what I'm supposed to look like!

Once you reveal your temple as God intended, take a moment to reflect on your journey. Remember your thought patterns and habits when you started. Look how much different you are now. Would you want to go back to the old you?

Your view of life will radically change. God will go from being thought of once in a while to the center of your life. Your sinful nature (with help from the devil) currently thinks this will be restricting and take the fun out of life. The exact opposite is true. **You will experience a freedom and peace of mind you never thought possible.**

This dramatic change, not only physically, but in spirit, will make others in awe of you. You will shine, and they will want to be like you. **Share.**

"Never give in—never, never, never, never, in nothing great or small, large or petty, never give in except to convictions of honor and good sense. Never yield to force; never yield to the apparently overwhelming might of the enemy."

Winston Churchill, in a speech given on October 29, 1941

Do not give in to the devil. He may appear overwhelming at times but he is not. In the game of weight loss the star player (God) is on your team. He wants to play but cannot unless you allow him into the game. If you use the abilities God has given you, and allow him in, he will use his supernatural talents and you will most certainly win. If you keep him on the sidelines, you will lose. The choice is yours.

"No one ever said at the end of his days; I have read my bible too much, I have thought of God too much, I have prayed too much, I have been too careful with my soul"
J.C. Ryle

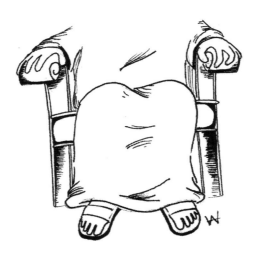

21

Standing Before God

The moment of truth.

Some day we will all have to stand before God and give an accounting of our life. There is nothing you can do about the past, but the present is in your hands. I don't know about you but when my turn comes, I want God to be able to say that once I figured out how to care for his temple, I was not perfect, but I did my best.

Following are two very powerful visualizations. Do them one right after the other. Notice the extreme contrast in emotions you feel.

Visualization – Standing Before God (as you are now)

Imagine you are standing before God. God is sitting on his throne in all his glory. There are angels and saints around God. All eyes are on you.

He asks you why you abused the temple he gave you. He says you know you could have asked for his help but you didn't and he wants to know why. He says your decision to abuse your temple inspired others not to follow Christ. He says these "others" saw you as preaching one thing and doing another. Imagine the shame you feel.

Visualization – Standing Before God (with your temple revealed)

Imagine you are standing before God. God is sitting on his throne in all his glory. There are angels and saints all around God. All of them are looking at you and smiling. God is smiling approvingly and is so proud of you. He says because you won the weight loss game, your example helped countless others care for their temples. **He says your example inspired others who were lost to become followers of Christ.**

Imagine how good you feel. Your choice to put God first in your life transformed you and countless others.

What if you kept these visualizations in mind whenever you were tempted? Would you win more battles, and ultimately the game?

"In conclusion, be strong in the Lord [be empowered through your union with Him]; draw your strength from Him [that strength which His boundless might provides]. Put on God's whole armor [the armor of a heavy-armed soldier which God supplies], that you may be able successfully to stand up against [all] the strategies and deceits of the devil."
Ephesians 6:10-11 (Amplified Bible)

"There are only two ways to live your life. One is as though nothing is a miracle. The other is as though everything is a miracle."
Albert Einstein

Listing of Visualizations

If you haven't started, get going!

The more you put into the visualizations, the more you'll get out of them. Use as many senses as you can. By doing the following, you'll see how much detail you already put into visualizations.

Go into your memory and think of a much cherished pleasant memory. Focus on the memory. What do you see? What do you hear? What do you smell? Do you feel hot or cold? Is it light or dark? What are the colors you see? What do you touch? It's amazing the detail we can recall.

As you practice the visualizations try to incorporate details such as these. The more you practice the more effective they will become.

Visualization – Waking Up

This is a great visualization to do each morning as soon as you wake up, while you are still in bed.

Imagine you just woke up from a good nights sleep. You look at the foot of your bed. Standing there is Jesus.

His clothing is radiant; it's like the sun is shining behind him. He is looking at you with a beautiful loving smile. His eyes sparkle. He stretches his arms out to you and says, "I have made this day, let's be happy and enjoy it!"

Kitchen

Go into your kitchen and find something healthy to eat, like a piece of fruit. Set it on the counter in front of you.

Imagine Jesus is standing right next to you. He is smiling at you like a parent smiles at his/her child. Look into his eyes and see all the love he has for you.

Pick up the fruit. Look at it closely, noticing its texture. Smell the fruit and enjoy its fragrant aroma. Now, look into his eyes and say as if this was the only food you would eat today "Thank you Lord, for this nourishment."

Turn away and set the fruit down. Pick up the fruit again and do it again. Repeat this 10 times.

After you have done this, go over to your cupboard and pick out some junk food. Set it on the same spot on the counter that you had the fruit.

Imagine Jesus standing next to you just as before. Pick up the junk food. Look at it closely, notice its texture and smell it. Think about what this junk food will do to your body once you have eaten it. After you have done this turn to Jesus, and look him in the eye and say, "Thank you for this nourishment." Were you able to do this? The more intense your visualization of Jesus the more likely you are not to want to touch the junk food.

Eating with the 5000

Imagine you are with Jesus and the 5000 when he fed them the fish and bread.

Feel the warmth of the sun on your skin, notice the smell of the water nearby. Feel the refreshing breeze in your hair.

Imagine the food you are eating was miraculously prepared by Jesus.

Look around you and notice other people in the crowd. You are seated near the feet of Jesus. As you eat each bite look up at Jesus and thank him for the nourishment.

Eating with Jesus
FOCUS ON JESUS. Do what I mentioned earlier, giving thanks for each bite. Imagine Jesus sitting across from you watching as you eat. If you are in a place where you can say it out loud do so, otherwise say it in your head.

At the Lord's Feet
The following visualization is really powerful, it can be extremely intense. You may want to do this in private. It alone can create an intense desire to want to care for your body. If you are able to, do this visualization kneeling by the side of your bed.

Imagine you are kneeling at the foot of a cross. You are so close to the cross you can touch it. You notice the grain in the wood and how rough the cutting is. You reach out and touch a sliver of wood that is sticking out from the cross with your finger. It is so sharp it pricks your finger.

Your gaze now shifts up the length of the cross.

Looking down at you is Jesus, dying on the cross. You can see everything, the spikes in his feet and hands, the crown of thorns. You hear his labored breathing, and see the blood coming from his wounds. You look at his face and can see sweat on his chin. Your gaze moves up his face and you see where the thorns are piercing the skin on his forehead. You can see droplets of blood forming where the thorns pierce the skin. You drop your head and gaze at the ground. A droplet of sweat hits you on the back of the neck. You look up again and Jesus is staring at you with his piercing eyes, they seem to look right through you. The look on his face is a combination of pain and love… for you. He says, "I am doing this, for you, take care of my Father's temple named (your name) for me."

You respond, "I will take care of this temple, my Lord and Savior, Jesus Christ."

The Mirror (As You Are Now)

Take a good look at yourself in the mirror. Notice in detail the excess weight on your body.

Imagine standing behind you is your child (ren) as adults, in the same physical shape.

Imagine behind your children a line of thousands of people, people as far as your eyes can see, all in the same physical shape as you are. These are your descendants for generations to come.

Statistics say if you do nothing about your temple this is the legacy you will leave. Do you like what you see?

The Mirror (Your Temple As God Intended)

Look at yourself in the mirror, not as you are but with the slim fit temple God intended you to have. Notice in detail how beautiful your temple is.

Imagine standing behind you are your child (ren) as adults slim and fit. Behind them is the line of thousands of descendants all looking slim and fit. They are all smiling at you, thanking you for the example you set for them. You can hear them saying "Thank you (your name)." If you allow God to help you become slim and fit, this is the likely legacy you will leave.

As you are aware, there are other people that look to you as a role model who are not related to you.

Neighbor kids, co-workers, friends etc. Often we are not even aware of how much influence we have on them. If you don't have children of your own, imagine some of these people in the mirror visualizations, with their descendants standing behind them.

Grocery Store

Imagine you have just entered your favorite grocery store. Guess who will be pushing your shopping cart? **Jesus.**

Imagine Jesus telling you how much he loves you and how proud he is of how you are cleaning up your temple.

Imagine walking each aisle of the store and putting the groceries in the cart. As you walk down the aisle that contains your greatest junk food temptations how do you feel? Can you put any junk food in the cart when Jesus is with you? **Do you think the devil is getting a little upset now that you have a new shopping buddy?**

Want to add a little muscle to your visualizing? When I am feeling especially weak I imagine Jesus showing up with the troops. If you are a Christian you know that God has sent angels to help watch over us and protect us. Why not imagine that a couple of warrior angels in battle gear each carrying a spear are with you to help protect you from the devil.

Walking On Water to Jesus

Imagine you are standing on the edge of a dock. The surface of the lake is only a few inches from the top of the dock. It's a beautiful sunny day with a few wispy clouds in the sky.

You are looking out across a peaceful serene lake. The water is so still it looks like glass. You can see the reflection of the clouds on the surface of the lake. On the other side of the lake is nothing but woods, it is so beautiful. You can hear the birds singing in the trees behind you.

You look across the lake towards the other shore and see someone standing, yes standing, in the middle of the lake. Standing on the surface of the lake is Jesus!

His face is glowing, he has a brilliant smile. His eyes are a clear blue and look as if beams of light are radiating from them. His robe is a brilliant white and his arms are outstretched….towards you.

He says, "Gaze into my eyes and come to me." You focus on his eyes….and step off the dock. You are standing on water! As you start to walk towards him you can feel the surface of the water on the bottom of your feet. You know if you divert your gaze from his eyes you will sink.

This is one of my favorite visualizations. It is fascinating to me the yearning to reach him that comes over me each time I do this visualization.

When I first started doing this I would not get very far before I would look at the lake and sink. As I've continued my journey I keep getting closer but have not made it all the way to his outstretched arms.

I was blown away one day while doing this visualization. When I reached a certain point in my walk to him something amazing happened. While gazing into his eyes they began to change! I was mesmerized as I watched them change from the clear blue with beams of light to a deep black with spiraling galaxies in each eye. I have found that each time I have done this visualization since, this change occurs at the same point in my journey to him.

Food Choice - Jesus vs. Devil

If you find yourself looking at a choice of junk food and nourishment and you're struggling, try this.

Jesus and the devil are standing in front of you.

Imagine Jesus is standing their holding the healthy food out to you. He is smiling at you, expecting you to make the right choice.

Imagine the devil is standing next to him holding the junk food out to you. The devil has a sly look and blazing red eyes.

Jesus says to you, "It's your choice."

Visualization – Devil Food Fight

Imagine you are standing in front of your pantry. Focus on a package of whatever food you craved most recently.

What are the words you thought that convinced you to starting to eat that food? Do these same words come to mind each time you are going to eat something you shouldn't?

Imagine picking up some of this food in your hand.

To your side is a door that is open just a crack, the devil is looking at you through the crack. He is sneering at you and laughing. Imagine throwing the food and as it splatters on the devil's face say out loud with a firm voice, **"NO CRACKS!"**

Repeat this with each food you crave.

Visualization – Standing Before God (as you are now)

Imagine you are standing before God.

God is sitting on his throne in all his glory. There are angels and saints around God. All eyes are on you.

He asks you why you abused the temple he gave you. He says you know you could have asked for his help but you didn't and he wants to know why. He says your decision to abuse your temple inspired others not to follow Christ.

He says these "others" saw you as preaching one thing and doing another.

Imagine the shame you feel.

Visualization – Standing Before God (with your temple revealed)

Imagine you are standing before God.

God is sitting on his throne in all his glory. There are angels and saints all around God. All of them are looking at you and smiling.

God is smiling approvingly and is so proud of you. He says because you won the weight loss game, your example helped countless others care for their temples. He says your example inspired others who were lost to become followers of Christ. Imagine how good you feel. Your choice to put God first in your life transformed you and countless others.

What if you kept these visualizations in mind whenever you were tempted? Would you win more battles, and ultimately the game?

List of Affirmations

Don't just think it, say it!

Words are important; they are part of your armor to successfully stand up against the devil. Pick out several affirmations or create your own. Memorize them and say them to yourself periodically throughout the day.

God is everywhere.

God is my comfort......not food.

I am dead to the sin of gluttony.

Everything I do, I do before God.

I will pray like God is coming today, I'll care for my temple like I'll live forever.

When tempted by the devil I will focus on God.

I will follow Jesus.

I am remodeling my temple for the Holy Spirit.

I will approach God with the heart of a child.

I am setting the standard for thousands who will follow me.

Everything I think and do today is an offering to God.

I will play the game of weight loss with God on my team.

When tempted I will make sure God is in the game.

Jesus always goes shopping with me.

Whenever I eat out I take Jesus as my guest.

My temple belongs to God.

My children's future health depends on my eating right.

My children are more important than stuffing myself.

Jesus is my guide through the weight loss wilderness.

I will take care of God's temple.

I will not dump garbage in God's temple.

Losing weight is an opportunity given to me by God, to grow and mature in my faith.

God is behind me every inch of the way.

Jesus is my weight loss buddy.

I am always eating for more than one; it's not just about me.

Thank you Lord, for this nourishment.

I am always aware of God's presence.

I am remodeling God's temple.

I am leaving a legacy of weight loss.

With God's help I am mastering the art of resisting temptation.

List of Bible Verses

"Put God in charge of your work, then what you've planned will take place."
Proverbs 16:3 (The Message)

"My choice is you God, first and only, And now I find I'm your choice!"
Psalm 16:5 (The Message)

"God's angels set up a circle of protection around us while we pray."
Psalm 34:7 (The Message)

"I can do all things through Christ who strengthens me."
Philippians 4:13 (NKJV)

"Day and night I'll stick with God; I've got a good thing going and I'm not letting go."
Psalm 16:8 (The Message)

".......All things can be (are possible) to him who believes!"
Mark 9:23 (Amplified Bible)

"God is our refuge and strength, a very present help in trouble, therefore we will not fear....."
Psalm 46:1-2 (NKJV)

"Trust God from the bottom of your heart; Don't try to figure out everything on your own. Listen for God's voice in everything you do, everywhere you go; he's the one who will keep you on track."
Proverbs 3:5-6 (The Message)

Morning Prayer

O Lord, Thank you for this beautiful day! I love you and will follow you all day long. Please stay in my thoughts through out this day. Thank you for helping me to reveal this temple, so I may use it to shine and glorify your great name.

Amen

Evening Prayer

O Lord, Thank you for being with me and watching over me this day! Please keep me in your loving care as I sleep. I look forward with anticipation to awakening tomorrow morning and spending another beautiful day with you. I love you and thank you for all you are doing in my life.

Amen

A Personal Message From Daniel Wychor

You've just finished the action guide, now is the time to start taking action! So where do you start?

Be aware that the devil uses temptation all the time. Many people will be tempted to set aside this action guide and get started later, for some later will never come. Don't make that mistake!

The following five keys are critical to your success.

1) Present moment awareness

Successful people spend most of their time focused on the present, not daydreaming about the past or future. It is when you are daydreaming about the past or future that you often reach for "comfort foods" which is a nice way of saying the devil is tempting you. Being aware of what is happening is critical to weight loss success. To help keep you aware and keep you from turning into a food zombie remember to use....

2) Awareness Cues

Use anything that will help you stay focused (pictures, crosses, figurines, music, rings etc.) around the house, at work, in your car etc. to keep you on track.

3) Remember the power of your words

Remember, what you say can affect you in a negative or positive way. Pick out a few affirmations from those provided and memorize them or come up with your own. Start reciting them through out the day, especially at times when you know you are tempted.

4) Visualization

Remember that when you think of food the devil starts tempting. Start using the visualizations right away so you can stop him in his tracks. Remember, visualizing is a wonderful gift God has given you. If you choose not to use it, the devil will use it against you. **Please don't let that happen!**

5) Read your Bible with anticipation

The Bible is literally God's living word. I had no idea what this meant until I started doing this. Don't forget to read your Bible as if it were your favorite mystery novel, a book that you can't put down. Before you start, ask God for guidance, telling him you can't wait to see what he is going to reveal to you as you read. You'll be amazed at the insights he gives you.

Commit to reading two chapters a day, one in the morning and one at night. As you grow and mature in your faith, this will become a part of your day you won't want to miss!

As was discussed earlier, this isn't just about weight loss. What you learned here, when applied, will help you deal with temptation in other areas of your life as well.

And finally… **God of the Angel Armies wants you!**

Let yourself become a shining example for your family, friends, fellow Christians, and generations yet to come!

God Bless,

Dan

You Are Not Alone!

Go to our website at http://dannywy.com
There you'll find helpful articles, videos and partner
resources to help you on your journey.

Made in the USA
Middletown, DE
17 December 2017